MITOCHONDRIA

DIET

Fueling Vitality and Optimal Health

By

HELEN HOLLIS

Mitochondria diet

Table of contents

INTRODUCTION: UNLOCKING THE POWER OF MITOCHONDRIA

Welcome to the vibrant world of mitochondrial health! In these pages, we embark on a culinary journey that transcends mere recipes—it's a voyage toward vitality, resilience, and well-being. So, grab your apron, sharpen your chef's knife, and let's explore the fascinating realm of mitochondria—the tiny powerhouses within our cells.

The Mighty Mitochondria: A Brief Overview

Mitochondria, those inconspicuous cellular dynamos, play a starring role in our overall health. Think of them as the energy factories humming away behind the scenes, diligently converting nutrients into adenosine triphosphate (ATP)—the currency of life. Without mitochondria, our bodies would be akin to a symphony without its conductor.

But there's more to these microscopic marvels than meets the eye. Beyond energy production, mitochondria influence our metabolism, immune response, and even our aging process. They're like the backstage crew, ensuring the show runs smoothly while we bask in the spotlight.

Why the Mitochondria Diet Matters

The "Mitochondria Diet" isn't just another fad—it's a science-backed approach to nourishing these cellular workhorses. By optimizing our nutrition, we can enhance mitochondrial function, boost energy levels, and fortify our health fortress. Imagine feeling invigorated, mentally sharp, and ready to conquer each day—all thanks to the food on your plate.

What Awaits You in This Cookbook

1. **Nutrient-Rich Recipes:** From antioxidant-packed berries to omega-3-rich salmon, our recipes spotlight ingredients that fuel mitochondria.

Expect vibrant salads, hearty stews, and guilt-free desserts—all designed to support cellular vitality.

2. **The Three-Week Plan:** We've crafted a practical three-week meal plan that gently nudges your mitochondria toward optimal performance. It's not a crash diet; it's a sustainable lifestyle shift.

3. **Kitchen Alchemy:** Learn how to transform everyday ingredients into potent elixirs for your cells. Discover the magic of spices, herbs, and superfoods that ignite mitochondrial sparks.

4. **Beyond the Plate**: It's not all about food. We delve into sleep hygiene, stress management, and movement—because holistic well-being extends beyond the kitchen.

A Culinary Adventure Awaits

Whether you're a seasoned home cook or a kitchen novice, this cookbook invites you to savor each bite with intention. Let's celebrate the synergy of flavors, the joy of nourishment, and the whisper of mitochondria humming their gratitude.

So, turn the page, ignite your stove, and let's cook up a healthier you—one mitochondrion at a time.

CHAPTER ONE : ESSENTIAL NUTRIENTS FOR MITOCHONDRIAL VITALITY

1. Antioxidants

Mitochondria are susceptible to oxidative stress, which can impair their function. Antioxidants help neutralize free radicals and protect these cellular powerhouses.

Include:

L-ascorbic acid: Found in citrus natural products, strawberries, and ringer peppers.

Vitamin E: Abundant in nuts, seeds, and spinach.

Selenium: Present in Brazil nuts, seafood, and whole grains.

2. B Vitamins

B vitamins play a crucial role in energy production and mitochondrial health.

Incorporate:

B1 (Thiamine): Whole grains, legumes, and pork.

B2 (Riboflavin): Dairy products, almonds, and leafy greens.

B3 (Niacin): Chicken, fish, and peanuts.

3. Coenzyme Q10 (CoQ10)

CoQ10 is like a spark plug for mitochondria. It aids ATP production and supports overall function.

Sources include:

- Fatty fish (salmon, mackerel)
- Organ meats (liver, heart)
- Spinach and broccoli

4. Magnesium

Magnesium is a multitasker—it activates enzymes involved in ATP synthesis and maintains mitochondrial integrity.

Get your dose from:

- Leafy greens (spinach, kale)
- Nuts (almonds, cashews)
- Whole grains

5. Omega-3 Fatty Acids

These healthy fats enhance mitochondrial efficiency and reduce inflammation.

Look for:

- Fatty fish (salmon, sardines)
- Flaxseeds and chia seeds
- Walnuts

Recipes to Boost Mitochondrial Health

1. Berry Bliss Smoothie:

  - Blend blueberries, spinach, almond milk, and a dash of ground flaxseed.

  - Rich in antioxidants and omega-3s.

2. Quinoa Salad with Avocado:

  - Combine cooked quinoa, avocado, cherry tomatoes, and fresh herbs.

  - Packed with magnesium and healthy fats.

3. Salmon and Broccoli Bake:

  - Roast salmon fillets with garlic, lemon, and broccoli.

  - CoQ10 and omega-3 goodness.

CHAPTER TWO

BREAKFAST BOOSTERS

Certainly! Let's kick off the "Breakfast Boosters" section with some energizing recipes to fuel your mornings. These dishes are designed to kickstart your day and support your mitochondria.

1. BERRY CHIA BREAKFAST BOWL

DESCRIPTION:

A vibrant and nutrient-packed bowl featuring antioxidant-rich berries, omega-3-loaded chia seeds, and creamy yogurt. It resembles an explosion of daylight in a bowl!

Prep Time: 10 minutes

Cook Time: 0 minutes

Servings: 2

INGREDIENTS:

- 1 cup blended berries (blueberries, raspberries, strawberries)
- 2 tablespoons chia seeds
- 1 cup Greek yogurt (or plant-based yogurt for a vegan option)
- 1 tablespoon honey or maple syrup (adjust to taste)
- Cut almonds or granola for fixing (discretionary)

INSTRUCTIONS:

1. In a bowl, mix the chia seeds with the yogurt. Let it sit for 5 minutes to allow the chia seeds to absorb some liquid.

2. Layer the yogurt-chia mixture with the mixed berries.

3. Sprinkle honey or maple syrup over the top.

4. Sprinkle with sliced almonds or granola for added crunch.

5. Dive in and enjoy the berrylicious goodness!

NUTRITIONAL INFORMATION (PER SERVING):

- Calories: 220
- Protein: 12g.
- Carbohydrates: 30g
- Healthy Fats: 7g
- Fiber: 8g

2. AVOCADO AND SPINACH OMELET

DESCRIPTION:

A protein-packed omelet infused with the goodness of creamy avocado and nutrient-rich spinach. It's a green powerhouse to fuel your morning.

Prep Time: 10 minutes
Cook Time: 5 minutes
Servings: 1

INGREDIENTS:

- 2 large eggs
- 1/2 ripe avocado, sliced

- Handful of fresh spinach leaves
- Salt and pepper to taste
- Olive oil or butter for cooking

INSTRUCTIONS:

1. Crack the eggs into a bowl, season with salt and pepper, and whisk until well combined.

2. Heat a non-stick skillet over medium heat and add a drizzle of olive oil or a pat of butter.

3. Pour the beaten eggs into the skillet, swirling to create an even layer.

4. Arrange the avocado slices and spinach leaves on one half of the omelet.

5. Fold the other half over the filling and cook for 2-3 minutes until set.

6. Gently slide the omelet onto a plate and serve hot.

NUTRITIONAL INFORMATION (PER SERVING):

- Calories: 320

- Protein: 18g

- Carbohydrates: 12g

- Fiber: 7g

- Healthy Fats: 24g

3. NUTTY QUINOA PORRIDGE

DESCRIPTION:

A warm and comforting quinoa porridge infused with nutty flavors, sweet dried fruits, and a hint of cinnamon. It's like a cozy hug for your mitochondria.

Prep Time: 10 minutes

Cook Time: 20 minutes

Servings: 2

INGREDIENTS:

- 1 cup cooked quinoa (cooked according to package instructions)
- 1 cup unsweetened almond milk (or any milk of your choice)
- 1/4 cup chopped dried apricots or raisins
- 2 tablespoons chopped walnuts or almonds
- 1 teaspoon ground cinnamon
- Sprinkle honey or maple syrup (optional)

INSTRUCTIONS:

1. In a pot, consolidate the cooked quinoa and almond milk.

2. Stir in the chopped dried apricots or raisins.

3. Simmer over low heat for about 15-20 minutes, stirring occasionally, until the mixture thickens to a porridge consistency.

4. Remove from heat and stir in the chopped nuts and ground cinnamon.

5. Sprinkle honey or maple syrup if desired.

6. Serve warm and enjoy the nutty goodness!

NUTRITIONAL INFORMATION (PER SERVING):

- Calories: 280
- Protein: 8g
- Carbohydrates: 45g
- Fiber: 6g
- Healthy Fats: 9g

4. GREEN SMOOTHIE BOWL

DESCRIPTION:

A refreshing and nutrient-packed green smoothie bowl that combines leafy greens, tropical fruits, and a sprinkle of superfoods. It's like a morning hug for your mitochondria.

Prep Time: 5 minutes
Cook Time: 0 minutes
Servings: 1

INGREDIENTS:

- 1 ripe banana

- 1 cup fresh spinach or kale

- 1/2 cup frozen pineapple chunks

- 1/2 cup unsweetened coconut water or almond milk

- Toppings: Chia seeds, sliced kiwi, and shredded coconut

INSTRUCTIONS:

1. In a blender, combine the banana, spinach or kale, frozen pineapple, and coconut water (or almond milk).

2. Blend until smooth and creamy.

3. Pour the green goodness into a bowl.

4. Top with chia seeds, sliced kiwi, and shredded coconut.

5. Grab a spoon and dive in!

NUTRITIONAL INFORMATION (PER SERVING):

- Calories: 250
- Protein: 5g
- Carbohydrates: 55g
- Fiber: 9g
- Healthy Fats: 2g

5. TURMERIC GOLDEN MILK OATMEAL

DESCRIPTION:

A cozy bowl of oatmeal infused with anti-inflammatory turmeric, warming spices, and creamy coconut milk. It's like a sunrise in a bowl!

Prep Time: 5 minutes
Cook Time: 10 minutes
Servings: 2

INGREDIENTS:

- 1 cup rolled oats

- 1 1/2 cups unsweetened coconut milk (or any milk of your choice)

- 1 teaspoon ground turmeric

- 1/2 teaspoon ground cinnamon

- Spot of dark pepper (to improve turmeric ingestion)

- Fixings: Cut bananas, hacked nuts, and a shower of honey

INSTRUCTIONS:

1. In a saucepan, combine the rolled oats, coconut milk, turmeric, cinnamon, and black pepper.

2. Cook over medium heat, stirring occasionally, until the oats are tender and creamy (about 8-10 minutes).

3. Eliminate the intensity and let it cool somewhat.

4. Serve in bowls and top with sliced bananas, chopped nuts, and a drizzle of honey.

5. Sip a cup of herbal tea alongside for the ultimate morning ritual.

NUTRITIONAL INFORMATION (PER SERVING):

- Calories: 280
- Protein: 6g
- Carbohydrates: 40g
- Fiber: 6g
- Healthy Fats: 12g

6. ENERGIZING MATCHA SMOOTHIE

DESCRIPTION:

A vibrant green smoothie featuring antioxidant-rich matcha, creamy avocado, and a hint of citrus. It resembles a harmony garden for your taste buds.

Prep Time: 5 minutes
Cook Time: 0 minutes
Servings: 1

INGREDIENTS:

- 1 ripe banana
- 1/2 ripe avocado
- 1 teaspoon matcha powder

- Juice of half a lime

- 1 cup unsweetened almond milk

- Ice cubes (optional)

INSTRUCTIONS:

1. Blend the banana, avocado, matcha powder, lime juice, and almond milk until smooth.

2. Add ice cubes if you prefer a chilled smoothie.

3. Pour into a glass and sip mindfully.

NUTRITIONAL INFORMATION (PER SERVING):

- Calories: 280

- Protein: 5g

- Carbohydrates: 45g

- Fiber: 10g

- Healthy Fats: 12g

7. OVERNIGHT CHIA PUDDING

DESCRIPTION:

A make-ahead delight that combines chia seeds, creamy coconut milk, and a hint of vanilla. It's like a dreamy dessert for breakfast.

Prep Time: 5 minutes (plus overnight soaking)
Cook Time: 0 minutes
Servings: 2

INGREDIENTS:

- 1/4 cup chia seeds

- 1 cup unsweetened coconut milk

- 1 teaspoon pure vanilla extract

- Fresh berries for topping

INSTRUCTIONS:

1. In a bowl, mix the chia seeds, coconut milk, and vanilla extract.

2. Cover and refrigerate overnight (or at least 4 hours) to allow the chia seeds to absorb the liquid.

3. Stir well before serving.

4. Top with fresh berries and savor the creamy goodness.

NUTRITIONAL INFORMATION (PER SERVING):

- Calories: 180
- Protein: 4g
- Carbohydrates: 12g
- Fiber: 10g
- Healthy Fats: 12g

8. ALMOND BUTTER BANANA TOAST

DESCRIPTION:

A simple yet satisfying toast that pairs creamy almond butter with ripe banana slices. It's a convenient solution for occupied mornings.

Prep Time: 5 minutes

Cook Time: 2 minutes

Servings: 1

INGREDIENTS:

- 1 slice whole-grain bread (toasted)

- 1 tablespoon almond butter

- 1 ripe banana, sliced

- A sprinkle of cinnamon

INSTRUCTIONS:

1. Toast the bread until golden brown.

2. Spread almond butter generously on the warm toast.

3. Arrange banana slices on top.

4. Dust with a pinch of cinnamon.

5. Enjoy your open-faced masterpiece!

NUTRITIONAL INFORMATION (PER SERVING):

- Calories: 280
- Protein: 7g
- Carbohydrates: 40g
- Fiber: 6g
- Healthy Fats: 12g

LUNCH

Certainly! Let's dive into the "Lunchtime Revitalizers" section. These recipes are designed to nourish your mitochondria and keep you energized throughout the day. Here are some revitalizing lunchtime options:

1. MEDITERRANEAN QUINOA SALAD

DESCRIPTION:

A vibrant salad bursting with Mediterranean flavors—quinoa, cherry tomatoes, cucumber, olives, and feta cheese. It's a nutrient-packed delight.

Prep Time: 15 minutes
Cook Time: 20 minutes (for quinoa)
Servings: 4

INGREDIENTS:

- 1 cup cooked quinoa (cooled)
- 1 cup cherry tomatoes, halved
- 1 cucumber, diced
- 1/2 red onion, thinly sliced
- 1/2 cup Kalamata olives, pitted
- 1/2 cup crumbled feta cheese
- Fresh parsley, chopped
- Lemon vinaigrette (olive oil, lemon juice, Dijon mustard, salt, and pepper)

INSTRUCTIONS:

1. In a large bowl, combine the cooked quinoa, cherry tomatoes, cucumber, red onion, olives, and feta cheese.

2. Drizzle with lemon vinaigrette and toss gently.

3. Garnish with fresh parsley.

4. Serve chilled or at room temperature.

NUTRITIONAL INFORMATION (PER SERVING):

- Calories: 280
- Protein: 10g
- Carbohydrates: 30g
- Fiber: 5g
- Healthy Fats: 14g

2. TURMERIC LENTIL SOUP

DESCRIPTION:

A warming soup infused with anti-inflammatory turmeric, protein-rich lentils, and a hint of coconut milk. Perfect for a cozy lunch.

Prep Time: 10 minutes
Cook Time: 30 minutes
Servings: 6

INGREDIENTS:

- 1 cup red lentils
- 1 onion, chopped

- 2 carrots, diced

- 2 garlic cloves, minced

- 1 teaspoon ground turmeric

- 4 cups vegetable broth

- 1 cup coconut milk

- Salt and pepper to taste

INSTRUCTIONS:

1. In a large pot, sauté the onion, carrots, and garlic until softened.

2. Add the lentils, turmeric, and vegetable broth.

3. Simmer for 25-30 minutes until the lentils are tender.

4. Mix in the coconut milk and season with salt and pepper.

5. Ladle into bowls and enjoy the golden goodness.

NUTRITIONAL INFORMATION (PER SERVING):

- Calories: 220

- Protein: 12g

- Carbohydrates: 30g

- Fiber: 8g

- Healthy Fats: 6g

3. Chickpea and Spinach Curry

DESCRIPTION:

A hearty curry featuring protein-packed chickpeas, vibrant spinach, and aromatic spices. A soothing bowl of goodness warms both body and soul.

Prep Time: 15 minutes

Cook Time: 25 minutes

Servings: 4

INGREDIENTS:

- 1 can (15 oz) chickpeas, drained and rinsed
- 1 onion, finely chopped
- 2 garlic cloves, minced
- 1 teaspoon ground cumin
- 1 teaspoon ground coriander
- 1/2 teaspoon ground turmeric
- 1/4 teaspoon cayenne pepper (adjust to taste)
- 1 can (14 oz) diced tomatoes
- 2 cups fresh spinach leaves
- Salt and pepper to taste
- Fresh cilantro for garnish

INSTRUCTIONS:

1. In a large skillet, sauté the chopped onion and minced garlic until fragrant.

2. Add the ground cumin, coriander, turmeric, and cayenne pepper. Stir well.

3. Pour in the diced tomatoes (with their juices) and chickpeas. Simmer for 15 minutes.

4. Add the fresh spinach leaves and cook until wilted.

5. Season with salt and pepper.

6. Serve over cooked brown rice or quinoa.

7. Garnish with fresh cilantro.

NUTRITIONAL INFORMATION (PER SERVING):

- Calories: 280.
- Healthy Fats: 5g
- Carbohydrates: 45g
- Fiber: 10g
- Protein: 12g

4. ROASTED VEGETABLE QUINOA BOWL

DESCRIPTION:

A colorful bowl featuring roasted veggies, fluffy quinoa, and a zesty lemon-tahini dressing. It's a balanced meal that satisfies both hunger and taste buds.

Prep Time: 20 minutes
Cook Time: 30 minutes
Servings: 4

INGREDIENTS:

- 1 cup cooked quinoa
- Assorted roasted vegetables (bell peppers, zucchini, eggplant, cherry tomatoes)
- 1/4 cup chopped fresh parsley
- Lemon-tahini dressing (whisk together tahini, lemon juice, garlic, salt, and water)

INSTRUCTIONS:

1. Arrange the cooked quinoa in bowls.
2. Top with roasted vegetables.
3. Drizzle with lemon-tahini dressing.
4. Sprinkle fresh parsley on top.
5. Enjoy the rainbow of flavors!

NUTRITIONAL INFORMATION (PER SERVING):

- Calories: 320
- Protein: 10g

- Carbohydrates: 50g
- Fiber: 8g
- Healthy Fats: 10g

5. Chickpea and Spinach Curry

DESCRIPTION:

A hearty curry featuring protein-packed chickpeas, vibrant spinach, and aromatic spices. A consoling bowl of goodness warms both body and soul.

Prep Time: 15 minutes
Cook Time: 25 minutes
Servings: 4

INGREDIENTS:

- 1 can (15 oz) chickpeas, drained and rinsed
- 1 onion, finely chopped
- 2 garlic cloves, minced
- 1 teaspoon ground cumin
- 1 teaspoon ground coriander
- 1/2 teaspoon ground turmeric
- 1/4 teaspoon cayenne pepper (adjust to taste)
- 1 can (14 oz) diced tomatoes
- 2 cups fresh spinach leaves
- Salt and pepper to taste
- Fresh cilantro for garnish

INSTRUCTIONS:

1. In a large skillet, sauté the chopped onion and minced garlic until fragrant.

2. Add the ground cumin, coriander, turmeric, and cayenne pepper. Stir well.

3. Pour in the diced tomatoes (with their juices) and chickpeas. Simmer for 15 minutes.

4. Add the fresh spinach leaves and cook until wilted.

5. Season with salt and pepper.

6. Serve over cooked brown rice or quinoa.

7. Garnish with fresh cilantro.

NUTRITIONAL INFORMATION (PER SERVING):

- Calories: 280   -Fiber: 10g

- Protein: 12g   -Healthy Fats: 5g

- Carbohydrates: 45g

6. ROASTED VEGETABLE QUINOA BOWL

DESCRIPTION:

A colorful bowl featuring roasted veggies, fluffy quinoa, and a zesty lemon-tahini dressing. It's a balanced meal that satisfies both hunger and taste buds.

Prep Time: 20 minutes
Cook Time: 30 minutes
Servings: 4

INGREDIENTS:

- 1 cup cooked quinoa

- Assorted roasted vegetables (bell peppers, zucchini, eggplant, cherry tomatoes)

- 1/4 cup chopped fresh parsley

- Lemon-tahini dressing (whisk together tahini, lemon juice, garlic, salt, and water)

INSTRUCTIONS:

1. Arrange the cooked quinoa in bowls.

2. Top with roasted vegetables.

3. Drizzle with lemon-tahini dressing.

4. Sprinkle fresh parsley on top.

5. Enjoy the rainbow of flavors!

NUTRITIONAL INFORMATION (PER SERVING):

- Calories: 320

- Protein: 10g

- Carbohydrates: 50g
- Fiber: 8g
- Healthy Fats: 10g

7. MEDITERRANEAN STUFFED BELL PEPPERS

DESCRIPTION:

Colorful bell peppers stuffed with a flavorful mixture of quinoa, chickpeas, sun-dried tomatoes, and fresh herbs. It's a wholesome and satisfying lunch.

Prep Time: 20 minutes
Cook Time: 30 minutes
Servings: 4

INGREDIENTS:

- 4 large bell peppers (any color)
- 1 cup cooked quinoa
- 1 can (15 oz) chickpeas, drained and rinsed
- 1/2 cup sun-dried tomatoes, chopped
- 1/4 cup fresh parsley, chopped
- 1 teaspoon dried oregano
- Salt and pepper to taste
- Olive oil for drizzling

INSTRUCTIONS:

1. Preheat the oven to 375°F (190°C).

2. Remove the tops the chime peppers and eliminate the seeds.

3. In a bowl, mix the cooked quinoa, chickpeas, sun-dried tomatoes, parsley, oregano, salt, and pepper.

4. Stuff each bell pepper with the quinoa mixture.

5. Drizzle with olive oil.

6. Place the stuffed peppers in a baking dish and cover with foil.

7. Bake for 25 minutes, then remove the foil and bake for an additional 5 minutes.

8. Serve hot and enjoy the Mediterranean goodness.

NUTRITIONAL INFORMATION (PER SERVING):

- Calories: 280

- Protein: 12g

- Carbohydrates: 45g

- Fiber: 10g

- Healthy Fats: 6g

8. ASIAN-INSPIRED EDAMAME SALAD

DESCRIPTION:

A refreshing salad featuring protein-rich edamame, crunchy veggies, and a sesame-ginger dressing. It's a delightful fusion of flavors.

Prep Time: 15 minutes
Cook Time: 5 minutes (for edamame)
Servings: 4

INGREDIENTS:

- 2 cups cooked edamame (shelled)
- 1 red bell pepper, thinly sliced
- 1 cucumber, diced

- 1 carrot, julienned
- 2 green onions, sliced
- Sesame seeds for garnish
- Dressing: Whisk together soy sauce, rice vinegar, sesame oil, grated ginger, and a touch of honey.

INSTRUCTIONS:

1. In a large bowl, combine the cooked edamame, bell pepper, cucumber, carrot, and green onions.
2. Drizzle with the sesame-ginger dressing and toss gently.
3. Sprinkle sesame seeds on top.
4. Serve chilled and savor the Asian flavors.

NUTRITIONAL INFORMATION (PER SERVING):

- Calories: 220
- Protein: 14g
- Carbohydrates: 25g
- Fiber: 8g
- Healthy Fats: 8g

9. *THAI-INSPIRED PEANUT NOODLE SALAD*

DESCRIPTION:

A zesty noodle salad featuring whole wheat noodles, crunchy veggies, and a creamy peanut dressing. It's a burst of Thai flavors in every bite.

Prep Time: 20 minutes
Cook Time: 10 minutes (for noodles)
Servings: 4

INGREDIENTS:

- 8 oz whole wheat noodles (such as udon or soba)

- 1 red bell pepper, thinly sliced

- 1 cup shredded purple cabbage

- 1 carrot, julienned

- 1/2 cup edamame (shelled)

- Fresh cilantro and chopped peanuts for garnish

- Dressing: Whisk together peanut butter, soy sauce, lime juice, honey, and a dash of sriracha.

INSTRUCTIONS:

1. Cook the noodles according to package instructions. Rinse with cold water and drain.

2. In a large bowl, combine the cooked noodles, bell pepper, cabbage, carrot, and edamame.

3. Drizzle with the peanut dressing and toss well.

4. Garnish with fresh cilantro and chopped peanuts.

5. Serve chilled or at room temperature.

NUTRITIONAL INFORMATION (PER SERVING):

- Calories: 320   - Healthy Fats: 10g
- Protein: 12g
- Carbohydrates: 50g
- Fiber: 8g

10. BALSAMIC GLAZED PORTOBELLO MUSHROOMS

DESCRIPTION:

Juicy portobello mushrooms marinated in balsamic vinegar and roasted to perfection. Serve them over a bed of quinoa or alongside a green salad.

Prep Time: 10 minutes
Cook Time: 20 minutes
Servings: 4

INGREDIENTS:

- 4 large portobello mushrooms, cleaned and stems removed
- 1/4 cup balsamic vinegar
- 2 tablespoons olive oil
- 2 garlic cloves, minced
- Salt and pepper to taste
- Fresh parsley for garnish

INSTRUCTIONS:

1. Preheat the oven to 375°F (190°C).
2. In a small bowl, whisk together the balsamic vinegar, olive oil, minced garlic, salt, and pepper.
3. Brush the portobello mushrooms with the marinade on both sides.
4. Place them on a baking sheet and roast for 15-20 minutes until tender.
5. Garnish with fresh parsley.

6. Serve warm and enjoy the umami goodness.

NUTRITIONAL INFORMATION (PER SERVING):

- Calories: 120

- Protein: 5g

- Carbohydrates: 10g

- Fiber: 3g

- Healthy Fats: 7g

DINNER

Certainly! Let's explore some delightful dinner recipes that will make your evenings special. From comforting casseroles to exotic flavors, these dishes are sure to satisfy your taste buds.

1. MAKEOVER HUSBAND'S DINNER DELIGHT

DESCRIPTION:

A revamped classic that your husband will adore! This casserole features extra-lean ground beef, tomato sauce, and a creamy cottage cheese layer. Serve it with whole wheat egg noodles for a wholesome meal.

Prep Time: 1 hour
Servings: 8
Calories per Serving: 382

INGREDIENTS:

- eight ounces uncooked whole wheat egg noodles
- 1 ½ pounds extra-lean ground beef (95% lean)
- 1 medium onion, chopped
- 1 medium green pepper, chopped
- 1 garlic clove, minced
- three cans (8 ounces each) tomato sauce
- 1 tablespoon sugar
- 1/8 teaspoon salt
- 1/8 teaspoon pepper
- 1 ½ cups 2% cottage cheese
- 4 ounces reduced-fat cream cheese
- ¼ cup reduced-fat sour cream
- 3 green onions, chopped
- ½ cup sharp cheddar cheese, shredded

INSTRUCTIONS:

1. Cook the whole wheat egg noodles according to package instructions. Drain and set aside.

2. In a skillet, brown the ground beef with onion, green pepper, and garlic.

3. Stir in the tomato sauce, sugar, salt, and pepper. Simmer for 10 minutes.

4. In a separate bowl, mix the cottage cheese, cream cheese, sour cream, and green onions.

5. Layer the cooked noodles, beef mixture, and cottage cheese mixture in a greased baking dish.

6. Top with shredded cheddar cheese.

7. Bake at 350°F (175°C) for 30 minutes or until bubbly and golden.

8. Let it rest for a few minutes before serving.

2. CREAMY CHICKEN DINNER DELIGHT

DESCRIPTION:

A slow-cooked chicken dish that's both creamy and flavorful. The combination of chicken thighs, potatoes, sun-dried tomatoes, and bacon creates a mouthwatering meal.

Prep Time: 4 hours 55 minutes
Servings: 12
Calories per Serving: 233

INGREDIENTS:

- 1 kilogram skinless chicken thigh fillets, sliced
- 3 washed potatoes (on the skin, 350g), diced into rough cubes
- 2 cloves garlic, minced
- 100 grams sun-dried tomatoes (in oil, oil drained)
- 100 grams bacon pieces, diced
- 1 red onion, diced chunky
- 8 button mushrooms, quartered
- 1 420-gram can cream of asparagus soup
- Salt and pepper to taste
- 300 milliliters light cream for cooking
- 1 cup broccoli florets, chopped

INSTRUCTIONS:

1. In a slow cooker, layer the chicken, potatoes, garlic, sun-dried tomatoes, bacon, onion, and mushrooms.

2. Pour in the cream of asparagus soup and light cream.

3. Season with salt and pepper.

4. Cook on low for 4 hours.

5. Add the broccoli florets and cook for an additional 55 minutes.

6. Serve hot and enjoy the creamy goodness.

3. LEMON HERB BAKED SALMON

DESCRIPTION:

A light and flavorful salmon dish infused with zesty lemon, fresh herbs, and a touch of garlic. It's a heart-healthy dinner that's ready in no time.

Prep Time: 10 minutes
Cook Time: 20 minutes
Servings: 4

INGREDIENTS:

- 4 salmon fillets (6 ounces each)
- Zest and juice of 1 lemon
- 2 tablespoons fresh dill, chopped

- 2 tablespoons fresh parsley, chopped

- 2 garlic cloves, minced

- Salt and pepper to taste

- Olive oil for drizzling

INSTRUCTIONS:

1. Preheat the oven to 375°F (190°C).

2. Put the salmon filets on a baking sheet fixed with material paper.

3. In a small bowl, mix the lemon zest, lemon juice, dill, parsley, minced garlic, salt, and pepper.

4. Sprinkle the herb mixture over the salmon.

5. Bake for 15-20 minutes or until the salmon is cooked through and flakes easily.

6. Serve with steamed asparagus or quinoa.

NUTRITIONAL INFORMATION (PER SERVING):

- Calories: 280

- Protein: 34g

- Carbohydrates: 2g

- Healthy Fats: 14g

4. RATATOUILLE STUFFED BELL PEPPERS

DESCRIPTION:

A twist on the classic ratatouille! These stuffed bell peppers are filled with a medley of eggplant, zucchini, tomatoes, and aromatic herbs. A sample of Provence in each nibble.

Prep Time: 20 minutes

Cook Time: 40 minutes

Servings: 6

INGREDIENTS:

- 6 large bell peppers (any color)

- 1 medium eggplant, diced

- 2 medium zucchini, diced

- 2 large tomatoes, diced

- 1 onion, chopped

- 2 garlic cloves, minced

- 2 tablespoons olive oil

- 1 teaspoon dried thyme

- Salt and pepper to taste

- Fresh basil for garnish

INSTRUCTIONS:

1. Preheat the oven to 375°F (190°C).

2. Remove the tops the chime peppers and eliminate the seeds.

3. In a skillet, sauté the onion and minced garlic in olive oil until softened.

4. Add the diced eggplant, zucchini, and tomatoes. Season with thyme, salt, and pepper.

5. Cook for 10 minutes until the vegetables are tender.

6. Stuff the bell peppers with the vegetable mixture.

7. Place them in a baking dish, cover with foil, and bake for 30 minutes.

8. Remove the foil and bake for an additional 10 minutes.

9. Garnish with fresh basil.

NUTRITIONAL INFORMATION (PER SERVING):

- Calories: 180

- Protein: 4g

- Carbohydrates: 25g

- Fiber: 8g

- Healthy Fats: 8g

5. LEMON HERB BAKED SALMON

DESCRIPTION:

A light and flavorful salmon dish infused with zesty lemon, fresh herbs, and a touch of garlic. It's a heart-healthy dinner that's ready in no time.

Prep Time: 10 minutes

Cook Time: 20 minutes

Servings: 4

INGREDIENTS:

- 4 salmon fillets (6 ounces each)

- Zest and juice of 1 lemon

- 2 tablespoons fresh dill, chopped

- 2 tablespoons fresh parsley, chopped

- 2 garlic cloves, minced

- Salt and pepper to taste

- Olive oil for drizzling

INSTRUCTIONS:

1. Preheat the oven to 375°F (190°C).

2. Put the salmon filets on a baking sheet fixed with material paper.

3. In a small bowl, mix the lemon zest, lemon juice, dill, parsley, minced garlic, salt, and pepper.

4. Sprinkle the herb mixture over the salmon.

5. Bake for 15-20 minutes or until the salmon is cooked through and flakes easily.

6. Serve with steamed asparagus or quinoa.

NUTRITIONAL INFORMATION (PER SERVING):

- Calories: 280
- Protein: 34g
- Carbohydrates: 2g
- Healthy Fats: 14g

6. RATATOUILLE STUFFED BELL PEPPERS

DESCRIPTION:

A twist on the classic ratatouille! These stuffed bell peppers are filled with a medley of eggplant, zucchini, tomatoes, and aromatic herbs. A sample of Provence in each nibble.

Prep Time: 20 minutes
Cook Time: 40 minutes
Servings: 6

INGREDIENTS:

- 6 large bell peppers (any color)
- 1 medium eggplant, diced
- 2 medium zucchini, diced
- 2 large tomatoes, diced
- 1 onion, chopped
- 2 garlic cloves, minced
- 2 tablespoons olive oil
- 1 teaspoon dried thyme
- Salt and pepper to taste
- Fresh basil for garnish

INSTRUCTIONS:

1. Preheat the oven to 375°F (190°C).

2. Remove the tops off the bell peppers and remove the seeds.

3. In a skillet, sauté the onion and minced garlic in olive oil until softened.

4. Add the diced eggplant, zucchini, and tomatoes. Season with thyme, salt, and pepper.

5. Cook for 10 minutes until the vegetables are tender.

6. Stuff the bell peppers with the vegetable mixture.

7. Place them in a baking dish, cover with foil, and bake for 30 minutes.

8. Remove the foil and bake for an additional 10 minutes.

9. Garnish with fresh basil.

NUTRITIONAL INFORMATION (PER SERVING):

- Calories: 180   - Healthy Fats: 8g
- Protein: 4g
- Carbohydrates: 25g
- Fiber: 8g

7. GREEK-INSPIRED LEMON HERB CHICKEN

DESCRIPTION:

A Mediterranean-inspired chicken dish marinated in lemon, garlic, and fresh herbs. Serve it with a side of roasted potatoes or a Greek salad for a complete meal.

Prep Time: 15 minutes (plus marinating time)
Cook Time: 30 minutes
Servings: 4

INGREDIENTS:

- 4 boneless, skinless chicken breasts
- Zest and juice of 1 lemon
- 2 tablespoons fresh oregano, chopped
- 2 tablespoons fresh rosemary, chopped
- 3 garlic cloves, minced
- Salt and pepper to taste
- Olive oil for cooking

INSTRUCTIONS:

1. In a bowl, mix the lemon zest, lemon juice, oregano, rosemary, minced garlic, salt, and pepper.

2. Place the chicken breasts in the marinade and refrigerate for at least 30 minutes (or up to 4 hours).

3. Heat olive oil in a skillet over medium intensity.

4. Cook the chicken breasts for about 6-8 minutes per side or until fully cooked.

5. Serve hot and garnish with additional lemon slices and fresh herbs.

NUTRITIONAL INFORMATION (PER SERVING):

- Calories: 220

- Protein: 34g

- Carbohydrates: 2g

- Healthy Fats: 8g

8. QUINOA-STUFFED ACORN SQUASH

DESCRIPTION:

A cozy and nutritious dish featuring roasted acorn squash halves filled with quinoa, cranberries, and toasted pecans. It's a delightful autumn-inspired dinner.

Prep Time: 20 minutes
Cook Time: 40 minutes
Servings: 4

INGREDIENTS:

- 2 acorn squash, halved and seeds removed
- 1 cup cooked quinoa
- 1/2 cup dried cranberries

- 1/2 cup toasted pecans, chopped

- 1 tablespoon maple syrup

- 1 teaspoon cinnamon

- Salt and pepper to taste

INSTRUCTIONS:

1. Preheat the oven to 375°F (190°C).

2. Place the acorn squash halves on a baking sheet, cut side up.

3. In a bowl, mix the cooked quinoa, cranberries, toasted pecans, maple syrup, cinnamon, salt, and pepper.

4. Fill each squash half with the quinoa mixture.

5. Cover with foil and prepare for 30 minutes.

6. Eliminate the foil and prepare for 10 extra minutes.

7. Serve warm and enjoy the autumn flavors.

NUTRITIONAL INFORMATION (PER SERVING):

- Calories: 280

- Protein: 6g

- Carbohydrates: 45g

- Fiber: 8g

- Healthy Fats: 10g

9. GREEK-INSPIRED LEMON HERB CHICKEN

DESCRIPTION:

A Mediterranean-inspired chicken dish marinated in lemon, garlic, and fresh herbs. Serve it with a side of roasted potatoes or a Greek salad for a complete meal.

Prep Time: 15 minutes (plus marinating time)
Cook Time: 30 minutes
Servings: 4

INGREDIENTS:

- 4 boneless, skinless chicken breasts
- Zest and juice of 1 lemon
- 2 tablespoons fresh oregano, chopped
- 2 tablespoons fresh rosemary, chopped
- 3 garlic cloves, minced
- Salt and pepper to taste
- Olive oil for cooking

INSTRUCTIONS:

1. In a bowl, mix the lemon zest, lemon juice, oregano, rosemary, minced garlic, salt, and pepper.

2. Place the chicken breasts in the marinade and refrigerate for at least 30 minutes (or up to 4 hours).

3. Heat olive oil in a skillet over medium intensity.

4. Cook the chicken breasts for about 6-8 minutes per side or until fully cooked.

5. Serve hot and garnish with additional lemon slices and fresh herbs.

NUTRITIONAL INFORMATION (PER SERVING):

- Calories: 220   - Healthy Fats: 8g
- Protein: 34g
- Carbohydrates: 2g

10.

QUINOA-STUFFED ACORN SQUASH

DESCRIPTION:

A cozy and nutritious dish featuring roasted acorn squash halves filled with quinoa, cranberries, and toasted pecans. It's a delightful autumn-inspired dinner.

Prep Time: 20 minutes
Cook Time: 40 minutes
Servings: 4

INGREDIENTS:

- 2 acorn squash, halved and seeds removed
- 1 cup cooked quinoa
- 1/2 cup dried cranberries
- 1/2 cup toasted pecans, chopped
- 1 tablespoon maple syrup
- 1 teaspoon cinnamon
- Salt and pepper to taste

INSTRUCTIONS:

1. Preheat the oven to 375°F (190°C).
2. Place the acorn squash halves on a baking sheet, cut side up.
3. In a bowl, mix the cooked quinoa, cranberries, toasted pecans, maple syrup, cinnamon, salt, and pepper.
4. Fill each squash half with the quinoa mixture.
5. Cover with foil and bake for 30 minutes.

6. Eliminate the foil and prepare for 10 extra minutes.

7. Serve warm and enjoy the autumn flavors.

NUTRITIONAL INFORMATION (PER SERVING):

- Calories: 280

- Protein: 6g

- Carbohydrates: 45g

- Fiber: 8g

- Healthy Fats: 10g

CHAPTER THREE

SNACKS AND SMOOTHIES

Certainly! Let's dive into some delicious snacks and smoothies to fuel your mitochondria. Here's the first recipe:

1. BERRY BLAST SMOOTHIE

DESCRIPTION:

A refreshing blend of antioxidant-rich berries to kickstart your day.

Prep Time: 5 minutes

Serving: 1

NUTRITIONAL INFORMATION:

- Calories: 180
- Protein: 8g
- Carbohydrates: 30g
- Fiber: 6g
- Healthy Fats: 4g

INGREDIENTS:

- one cup mixed berries (blueberries, raspberries, strawberries)
- 1 banana
- 1 cup spinach
- 1 tablespoon chia seeds
- 1 cup unsweetened almond milk
- Ice cubes (optional)

INSTRUCTIONS:

1. Mix all ingredients to a blender.

2. Blend until smooth.

3. Pour into a glass and enjoy!

2. GREEN GODDESS SMOOTHIE

DESCRIPTION:

A vibrant green blend packed with leafy greens and healthy fats.

Prep Time: 5 minutes

Serving: 1

NUTRITIONAL INFORMATION:

- Calories: 220
- Protein: 10g
- Carbohydrates: 20g
- Fiber: 8g
- Healthy Fats: 12g

INGREDIENTS:

- 1 cup kale or spinach
- 1 ripe avocado
- 1 tablespoon almond butter
- 1 cup unsweetened coconut water
- Juice of 1 lime
- Ice cubes (optional)

INSTRUCTIONS:

1. Blend all ingredients until smooth.

2. Pour into a glass and enjoy the green goodness!

3. Chia Berry Parfait

Description:

A parfait layered with chia pudding and fresh berries.

Prep Time: 10 minutes (plus chia pudding chilling time)
Serving: 1

NUTRITIONAL INFORMATION:

- Calories: 280

- Protein: 8g

- Carbohydrates: 35g

- Fiber: 12g

- Healthy Fats: 10g

INGREDIENTS:

- 2 tablespoons chia seeds

- 1 cup unsweetened almond milk

- one cup add berries (strawberries, blueberries, raspberries)

- 1 tablespoon chopped nuts (almonds, walnuts)

Instructions:

1. Mix chia seeds and almond milk. Refrigerate for at least two hours or overnight.

2. Layer chia pudding with berries in a glass.

3. Top with chopped nuts and enjoy!

4. TURMERIC GOLDEN MILK SMOOTHIE

DESCRIPTION:

A warming and anti-inflammatory blend with a hint of spice.

Prep Time: 5 minutes
Serving: 1

NUTRITIONAL INFORMATION:

- Calories: 200

- Protein: 6g

- Carbohydrates: 25g

- Fiber: 4g

- Healthy Fats: 8g

INGREDIENTS:

- 1 cup unsweetened almond milk

- 1 ripe banana

- 1 teaspoon ground turmeric

- 1/2 teaspoon ground cinnamon

- 1/4 teaspoon ground ginger

- Pinch of black pepper (to enhance turmeric absorption)

- 1 tablespoon honey or maple syrup if desire

INSTRUCTIONS:

1. Blend all ingredients until smooth.

2. Heat gently on the stovetop if you prefer a warm drink.

3. Sip and enjoy the golden goodness!

5. AVOCADO CHOCOLATE SMOOTHIE

DESCRIPTION:

Creamy and indulgent, this smoothie satisfies your sweet tooth.

Prep Time: 5 minutes

Serving: 1

NUTRITIONAL INFORMATION:

- Calories: 280
- Protein: 10g
- Carbohydrates: 30g
- Fiber: 10g
- Healthy Fats: 15g

INGREDIENTS:

- 1 ripe avocado

- 1 tablespoon unsweetened cocoa powder

- 1 cup unsweetened almond milk

- 1 tablespoon chia seeds

- 1 teaspoon vanilla extract

- Ice cubes (optional)

INSTRUCTIONS:

1. Blend all ingredients until creamy.

2. Add ice cubes if desired.

3. Pour into a glass and savor the chocolatey goodness!

6. MATCHA MINT SMOOTHIE

DESCRIPTION:

A refreshing blend with the goodness of matcha and a hint of mint.

Prep Time: 5 minutes

Serving: 1

NUTRITIONAL INFORMATION:

- Calories: 160
- Protein: 5g
- Carbohydrates: 20g
- Fiber: 4g
- Healthy Fats: 6g

INGREDIENTS:

- 1 teaspoon matcha powder

- 1 cup unsweetened coconut milk

- Handful of fresh mint leaves

- one tablespoon honey or agave syrup

- Ice cubes (optional)

INSTRUCTIONS:

1. Blend all ingredients until smooth.

2. Adjust sweetness to taste.

3. Garnish with mint leaves and enjoy the vibrant green drink!

7. COCONUT ALMOND BLISS SMOOTHIE

DESCRIPTION:

Creamy and nutty, this smoothie is a tropical treat.

Prep Time: 5 minutes

Serving: 1

NUTRITIONAL INFORMATION:

- Calories: 250
- Protein: 9g
- Carbohydrates: 20g
- Fiber: 6g
- Healthy Fats: 15g

INGREDIENTS:

- 1 cup unsweetened coconut milk

- 1 ripe banana

- 2 tablespoons almond butter

- 1 tablespoon shredded coconut

- Ice cubes (optional)

INSTRUCTIONS:

1. Blend all ingredients until smooth.

2. Garnish with extra shredded coconut.

3. Sip and transport yourself to a tropical paradise!

8. POMEGRANATE POWER SMOOTHIE

Description:

A vibrant red blend bursting with antioxidants.

Prep Time: 5 minutes
Serving: 1

NUTRITIONAL INFORMATION:

- Calories: 190
- Protein: 7g
- Carbohydrates: 25g
- Fiber: 5g
- Healthy Fats: 8g

INGREDIENTS:

- 1 cup pomegranate seeds (fresh or frozen)
- 1 cup unsweetened Greek yogurt
- 1 tablespoon honey
- 1/2 teaspoon vanilla extract
- Ice cubes (optional)

INSTRUCTIONS:

1. Blend pomegranate seeds, yogurt, honey, and vanilla until well combined.

2. Add ice cubes if desired.

3. Pour into a glass and enjoy the burst of flavor!

9. MINTY MATCHA ENERGY BITES

DESCRIPTION:

A snack that combines the power of matcha and the freshness of mint.

Prep Time: 15 minutes

Serving: Makes about 12 bites

NUTRITIONAL INFORMATION (PER BITE):

- Calories: 80
- Protein: 2g
- Carbohydrates: 10g
- Fiber: 2g
- Healthy Fats: 4g

INGREDIENTS:

- 1 cup rolled oats
- 1/2 cup almond butter
- 2 tablespoons matcha powder
- 1 tablespoon honey
- 1/4 cup chopped fresh mint leaves

INSTRUCTIONS:

1. Add all ingredients in a bowl until well mixed.

2. Roll into bite-sized balls.

3. Refrigerate for at least 30 minutes before enjoying.

10. COCOA AVOCADO MOUSSE

DESCRIPTION:

 A guilt-free dessert that combines the creaminess of avocado with the richness of cocoa.

Prep Time: 10 minutes
Chilling Time: 1 hour
Serving: 2

NUTRITIONAL INFORMATION (PER SERVING):

- Calories: 220

- Protein: 4g

- Carbohydrates: 20g

- Fiber: 8g

- Healthy Fats: 15g

INGREDIENTS:

- 1 ripe avocado
- 2 tablespoons unsweetened cocoa powder
- 2 tablespoons honey or maple syrup
- 1 teaspoon vanilla extract
- Pinch of sea salt

INSTRUCTIONS:

1. Scoop out the avocado flesh and blend it with cocoa powder, honey, vanilla, and salt until smooth.

2. Chill in the refrigerator for at least one hour.

3. Serve in small bowls or glasses and enjoy the velvety mousse!

MITOCHONDRIA DESSERT

Certainly! Let's explore some delightful "Mitochondrial Desserts" to satisfy your sweet cravings while supporting cellular health.

1. CHIA BERRY PARFAIT

DESCRIPTION:
 A parfait layered with chia pudding and fresh berries.

Prep Time:10 minutes (plus chia pudding chilling time)

Serving:1

NUTRITIONAL INFORMATION (PER SERVING):

- Calories: 280
- Protein: 8g
- Carbohydrates: 35g
- Fiber: 12g
- Healthy Fats: 10g

INGREDIENTS:

- 2 tablespoons chia seeds
- 1 cup unsweetened almond milk
- 1 cup add berries (strawberries, blueberries, raspberries)
- 1 tablespoon chopped nuts (almonds, walnuts)

INSTRUCTIONS:

1. Mix chia seeds and almond milk. Refrigerate for at least two hours or overnight.

2. Layer chia pudding with berries in a glass.

3. Top with chopped nuts and enjoy this wholesome treat!

2. AVOCADO CHOCOLATE MOUSSE

DESCRIPTION:

A guilt-free dessert that combines the creaminess of avocado with the richness of cocoa.

Prep Time:10 minutes

Chilling Time: 1 hour

Serving: 2

NUTRITIONAL INFORMATION (PER SERVING):

- Calories: 220

- Protein: 4g

- Carbohydrates: 20g

- Fiber: 8g

- Healthy Fats: 15g

INGREDIENTS:

- 1 ripe avocado

- 2 tablespoons unsweetened cocoa powder

- 2 tablespoons honey or maple syrup

- 1 teaspoon vanilla extract

- Pinch of sea salt

INSTRUCTIONS:

1. Scoop out the avocado flesh and blend it with cocoa powder, honey, vanilla, and salt until smooth.

2. Chill in the refrigerator for at least one hour.

3. Serve in small bowls or glasses and enjoy the velvety mousse!

3. COCONUT ALMOND BLISS BITES

DESCRIPTION:

Nutty and satisfying bites with a hint of coconut.

Prep Time: 15 minutes

Chilling Time: 30 minutes

Serving: Makes about 12 bites

NUTRITIONAL INFORMATION (PER BITE):

- Calories: 100

- Protein: 3g

- Carbohydrates: 10g

- Fiber: 2g

- Healthy Fats: 6g

INGREDIENTS:

- 1 cup unsweetened shredded coconut

- 1/2 cup almond flour

- 2 tablespoons coconut oil (melted)

- one tablespoon honey or agave syrup

- Pinch of sea salt

INSTRUCTIONS:

1. Mix shredded coconut, almond flour, melted coconut oil, honey, and salt in a bowl.

2. Roll into bite-sized balls.

3. Refrigerate for 30 minutes before enjoying.

4. BLUEBERRY CHIA JAM

DESCRIPTION:

A simple, no-sugar-added jam bursting with antioxidants.

Prep Time: 10 minutes

Cook Time: 20 minutes

Serving: Approximately 1 cup

NUTRITIONAL INFORMATION (PER TABLESPOON)

- Calories: 20
- Carbohydrates: 5g
- Fiber: 2g
- Healthy Fats: 0g

INGREDIENTS:

- 1 cup fresh or frozen blueberries
- 2 tablespoons chia seeds
- Juice of 1 lemon
- Water (as needed for desired consistency)

INSTRUCTIONS:

1. In a saucepan, combine blueberries and lemon juice. Simmer over low heat until berries soften.

2. Mash the berries with a fork or potato masher.

3. Stir in chia seeds and add water if needed.

4. Let it cool and thicken. Store in a glass container and refrigerate.

5. DARK CHOCOLATE AVOCADO TRUFFLES

DESCRIPTION:

Decadent truffles with a secret healthy twist.

Prep Time: 15 minutes

Chilling Time: 1 hour

Serving: Makes about 12 truffles

NUTRITIONAL INFORMATION (PER TRUFFLE):

- Calories: 80

- Protein: 2g

- Carbohydrates: 6g

- Fiber: 2g

- Healthy Fats: 6g

INGREDIENTS:

- 1 ripe avocado

- 1/4 cup unsweetened cocoa powder

- 2 tablespoons honey or maple syrup

- 1 teaspoon vanilla extract

- Pinch of sea salt

- Unsweetened destroyed coconut or cocoa powder for covering

INSTRUCTIONS:

1. Blend avocado, cocoa powder, honey, vanilla, and salt until smooth.

2. Chill the mixture for 30 minutes.

3. Roll into truffle-sized balls and coat with shredded coconut or cocoa powder.

4. Chill for another 30 minutes before serving.

6. RASPBERRY ALMOND THUMBPRINT COOKIES

DESCRIPTION:

Nutty cookies with a burst of raspberry goodness.

Prep Time: 20 minutes

Cook Time: 15 minutes

Serving: Makes about 12 cookies

NUTRITIONAL INFORMATION (PER COOKIE):

- Calories: 120

- Protein: 3g

- Carbohydrates: 10g

- Fiber: 2g

- Healthy Fats: 8g

INGREDIENTS:

- 1 cup almond flour

- 2 tablespoons coconut oil (melted)

- 2 tablespoons honey

- 1/4 cup raspberry jam (no added sugar)

1. Preheat the oven to 350°F (180°C).

2. Mix almond flour, melted coconut oil, and honey to form a dough.

3. Shape into small cookies and make a thumbprint in the center.

4. Fill each thumbprint with raspberry jam.

5. Prepare for 12-15 minutes until brilliant.

7. MATCHA COCONUT ENERGY BALLS

DESCRIPTION:

A bite-sized snack with the goodness of matcha and coconut.

Prep Time: 15 minutes

Chilling Time: 30 minutes

Serving: Makes about 12 energy balls

NUTRITIONAL INFORMATION (PER ENERGY BALL):

- Calories: 90

- Protein: 2g

- Carbohydrates: 10g

- Fiber: 2g
- Healthy Fats: 5g

INGREDIENTS:

- 1 cup unsweetened shredded coconut
- 2 tablespoons almond flour
- 1 tablespoon matcha powder
- two tablespoons honey or agave syrup
- Pinch of sea salt

INSTRUCTIONS:

1. Mix shredded coconut, almond flour, matcha powder, honey, and salt in a bowl.

2. Roll into energy ball-sized portions.

3. Refrigerate for 30 minutes before enjoying.

8. WALNUT DATE TRUFFLES

DESCRIPTION:

Nutty and naturally sweet truffles.

Prep Time: 20 minutes

Chilling Time: 1 hour

Serving: Makes about 12 truffles

NUTRITIONAL INFORMATION (PER TRUFFLE):

- Calories: 100   - Fiber: 2g

- Healthy Fats: 5g

- Protein: 2g

- Carbohydrates: 12g

INGREDIENTS:

- 1 cup walnuts
- 1 cup pitted dates
- 1 tablespoon unsweetened cocoa powder
- 1 teaspoon vanilla extract
- Unsweetened shredded coconut for coating

INSTRUCTIONS:

1. Blend walnuts, dates, cocoa powder, and vanilla until a sticky mixture forms.
2. Roll into truffle-sized balls.
3. Coat with shredded coconut.
4. Chill for an hour before serving.

9. BERRY AVOCADO POPSICLES

DESCRIPTION:

Refreshing popsicles with a creamy twist.

Prep Time:10 minutes
Freezing Time: 4 hours
Serving: Makes 6 popsicles

NUTRITIONAL INFORMATION (PER POPSICLE):

- Calories: 70

- Protein: 1g

- Carbohydrates: 10g

- Fiber: 2g

- Healthy Fats: 3g

INGREDIENTS:

- 1 ripe avocado

- 1 cup combined berries (blueberries, raspberries, strawberries)

- one tablespoon honey or agave syrup

- Juice of 1 lemon

INSTRUCTIONS:

1. Blend avocado, berries, honey, and lemon juice until smooth.

2. Pour into popsicle molds.

3. Freeze for at least four hours.

4. Enjoy these fruity, creamy treats!

10. CINNAMON APPLE CRISP

DESCRIPTION:

Warm, spiced apples topped with a crunchy oat crumble.

Prep Time: 15 minutes

Baking Time: 30 minutes

Serving: 4

NUTRITIONAL INFORMATION (PER SERVING):

- Calories: 180   - Healthy Fats: 4g
- Protein: 2g
- Carbohydrates: 35g
- Fiber: 5g

INGREDIENTS:

- 4 medium apples (peeled, cored, and sliced)
- 1 tablespoon lemon juice
- 1 teaspoon ground cinnamon
- 1/2 cup rolled oats
- 1/4 cup almond flour
- 2 tablespoons coconut oil (melted)
- 2 tablespoons honey or maple syrup

INSTRUCTIONS:

1. Preheat the oven to 350°F (180°C).

2. Toss apple slices with lemon juice and cinnamon. Place in a baking dish.

3. In a separate bowl, mix oats, almond flour, melted coconut oil, and honey.

4. Sprinkle the oat mixture over the apples.

5. Bake for 30 minutes or until the topping is golden and apples are tender.

6. Serve warm with a dollop of Greek yogurt or coconut whipped cream.

CHAPTER FOUR: WEEKEND WELLNESS MEALS

Certainly! Let's explore some delightful "Weekend Wellness Meals"

1. MEDITERRANEAN MEZZE PLATTER

DESCRIPTION: A colorful spread of Mediterranean-inspired appetizers.

COMPONENTS:
- Hummus
- Tzatziki
- Falafel
- Stuffed grape leaves (dolmas)
- Olives

- Pita bread or whole-grain crackers

Serve with: Fresh veggies and a glass of chilled white wine.

2. SLOW-COOKED COQ AU VIN

DESCRIPTION:

A classic French dish of chicken braised in red wine.

INGREDIENTS:

- Chicken thighs or drumsticks
- Red wine
- Pearl onions
- Mushrooms
- Bacon
- Garlic
- Thyme and bay leaves

Serve with: Crusty baguette or mashed potatoes.

3. INDIAN VEGETABLE BIRYANI

DESCRIPTION: Fragrant rice dish with spices, vegetables, and nuts.

Ingredients:

- Basmati rice

- Mixed veggies (carrots, peas, bell peppers)

- Saffron strands

- Cashews and raisins

- Garam masala

Serve with: Raita (yogurt sauce) and mango chutney.

4. JAPANESE OKONOMIYAKI

DESCRIPTION: Savoy cabbage pancakes with various toppings.

Ingredients:

- Cabbage

- Flour

- Eggs

- Shredded carrots

- Green onions

- Bonito flakes and okonomiyaki sauce

Serve with:Pickled ginger and a cold Japanese beer.

5. MEXICAN CHILES RELLENOS

DESCRIPTION: Stuffed poblano peppers in tomato sauce.

INGREDIENTS:

- Poblano peppers

- Cheese or minced meat filling

- Egg batter

- Tomato sauce

Serve with: Mexican rice and refried beans.

6. SPANISH PAELLA

DESCRIPTION:A vibrant rice dish loaded with saffron, seafood, and vegetables.

INGREDIENTS:

- Arborio rice

- Saffron threads

- Shrimp, mussels, and squid

- Bell peppers

- Tomatoes

- Chorizo (optional)

- **Serve with**: A glass of sangria and crusty bread.

7. THAI GREEN CURRY

DESCRIPTION: Fragrant and spicy curry with coconut milk, vegetables, and herbs.

INGREDIENTS:

- Green curry paste

- Coconut milk

- Mixed veggies (eggplant, bell peppers, zucchini)

- Thai basil and kaffir lime leaves

Serve with: Jasmine rice or rice noodles.

8. GREEK MOUSSAKA

DESCRIPTION: Layers of eggplant, spiced meat, and creamy béchamel sauce.

INGREDIENTS:

- Eggplant
- Ground lamb or beef
- Onion and garlic
- Cinnamon and nutmeg
- Tomato sauce
- Béchamel sauce

Serve with: Greek salad and warm pita bread.

9. BRAZILIAN FEIJOADA

DESCRIPTION:Hearty black bean stew with various meats.

INGREDIENTS:

- Black beans

- Pork shoulder, sausage, and bacon

- Onion, garlic, and bell peppers

- Orange slices (for garnish)

Serve with: White rice and farofa (toasted cassava flour).

10. ITALIAN TIRAMISU

DESCRIPTION: Classic dessert with layers of coffee-soaked ladyfingers and mascarpone cream.

INGREDIENTS:

- Ladyfingers

- Espresso or strong coffee

- Mascarpone cheese

- Cocoa powder

- Dark chocolate shavings

Serve chilled as a sweet finale!

3-WEEK "MITOCHONDRIAL RESET PLAN"

Week 1: Fueling Mitochondria

1. Day 1 (Monday):

Breakfast: Greek yogurt with berries and chia seeds.

Lunch: Quinoa salad with roasted veggies and avocado.

Dinner: Baked salmon with steamed broccoli and sweet potato.

2. Day 3 (Wednesday):

Breakfast: Spinach and mushroom omelet.

Lunch: Lentil soup with a side of mixed greens.

Dinner: Grilled chicken breast with asparagus and quinoa.

3. Day 5 (Friday):

Breakfast: Smoothie (spinach, banana, almond butter, and coconut milk).

Lunch: Chickpea salad with cucumber, tomatoes, and feta.

Dinner:Stir-fried tofu with bok choy and brown rice.

Week 2: Intermittent Fasting

1. Day 8 (Monday):

Breakfast: Black coffee or herbal tea (fasting until lunch).

Lunch: Lentil stew with a side of sautéed spinach.

Dinner: Grilled fish with roasted Brussels sprouts.

2. Day 10 (Wednesday):

Breakfast:Green tea (fasting until lunch).

Lunch: Quinoa and black bean salad.

Dinner: Zucchini noodles with pesto and grilled shrimp.

3. Day 12 (Friday):

Breakfast: Water with lemon (fasting until lunch).

Lunch:Chickpea and vegetable curry.

Dinner: Baked cod with cauliflower rice.

Week 3: Nutrient-Dense Meals

1. Day 15 (Monday):

Breakfast: Berry smoothie with spinach and hemp seeds.

Lunch:Spinach salad with grilled chicken and walnuts.

Dinner:Turkey meatballs with roasted eggplant.

2. Day 17 (Wednesday):

Breakfast:Avocado toast with poached eggs.

Lunch: Miso soup with seaweed and tofu.

Dinner: Beef stir-fry with broccoli and ginger.

3. Day 19 (Friday):

Breakfast: Fasting (water or herbal tea).

Lunch: Quinoa-stuffed bell peppers.

Dinner: Baked sweet potato with black beans and salsa.

1. Quality sleep:

- Focus on getting 7-9 hours of serene rest every evening.

- Make a quieting sleep time schedule: faint lights, stay away from screens, and practice unwinding methods.

- Sleep is when your body repairs and rejuvenates, including your mitochondria.

2. Stress Management:

- Chronic stress can impact mitochondrial function.

- Practice care, reflection, or profound breathing activities.

- Participate in exercises you appreciate to lessen feelings of anxiety.

3. Regular Movement:

- Exercise supports mitochondrial health by enhancing energy production.

- Aim for a mix of aerobic (cardio), strength training, and flexibility exercises.

- Track down development that gives you pleasure — whether it's moving, climbing, or yoga.

4. Sunshine and Vitamin D:

- Sun exposure helps your body produce vitamin D, which plays a role in mitochondrial function.

- Spend time outdoors, especially during sunny hours (safely, with sunscreen).

5. Cold Exposure (Cryotherapy):

- Cold showers or ice baths can activate brown fat and boost mitochondrial activity.

- Start gradually and consult a healthcare professional if you have any health concerns.

6. Intermittent Fasting (IF):

- You mentioned this earlier! IF can enhance mitochondrial efficiency.

- Consider a 16:8 fasting window (16 hours without food, 8-hour eating window).

7. Hydration:

- Proper hydration supports cellular processes, including mitochondrial function.

- Hold back nothing to 8 glasses of water day to day.

8. Social Connections:

- Meaningful relationships positively impact overall health.
- Spend time with loved ones, even virtually.

9. Mindful Eating:

- Chew slowly, savor your meals, and pay attention to hunger cues.
- Keep away from careless nibbling or profound eating.

10. Gratitude and Positivity:

- Cultivate a positive mindset.
- Practice gratitude—write down things you're thankful for each day.

Remember, vitality is a holistic journey. Listen to your body, adapt these tips to your lifestyle, and enjoy the process!

Conclusion: Nourishing from Within

Dear readers,

As we reach the final pages of our culinary journey through the world of mitochondria-friendly meals, I want to express my gratitude for joining me on this adventure. The "Mitochondria Diet: Fueling Vitality and Optimal Health" isn't just a collection of recipes—it's a celebration of life, energy, and the intricate dance of our cellular powerhouses.

What We've Discovered

We've explored vibrant breakfast boosters that kickstart our mornings with nutrient-packed smoothies. We've savored lunchtime revitalizers—nutrient-dense salads, soups, and stews that sustain us through busy afternoons. Our dinner delights have been wholesome, colorful, and brimming with flavors that nourish both body and spirit.

But this cookbook isn't only about food. It's tied in with embracing a comprehensive way to deal with imperativeness. So, let's recap the lifestyle tips that complement our

culinary creations:

1. Sleep Well: Remember, your mitochondria love a good night's rest. Prioritize sleep—it's when they repair, regenerate, and whisper secrets of energy.

2. Stress Less: Breathe deeply, find your calm, and let stress dissipate like morning mist. Your mitochondria thrive in a peaceful environment.

3. Move Joyfully: Whether it's a dance in the living room or a hike in the woods, movement fuels your cells. Let your body sway to its own rhythm.

4. Soak Up Sunshine: Vitamin D, like a warm embrace from the sun, supports

mitochondrial function. Step outside, feel the rays, and smile.

5. Intermittent Fasting: Give your mitochondria a break. Intermittent fasting invites them to tidy up, rearrange furniture, and optimize their energy factories.

6. Hydrate Mindfully: Water is life. Sip it consciously, and watch your cells dance in gratitude.

7. Connect: Laugh with friends, hug your loved ones, and share meals. Social bonds are the secret sauce of vitality.

8. Practice Gratitude: Each bite, each sunrise, each heartbeat—gratefulness infuses life with magic.

Beyond Recipes: A Symphony of Wellness

As you close this cookbook, remember that you're not just closing a book. You're stepping into a symphony—a harmonious blend of flavors, movement, and mindful living. Your mitochondria, those tireless conductors, are ready to lead the orchestra of your existence.

So, cook with love, eat with intention, and savor every moment. May your mitochondria hum with joy, and may your life be a delicious melody.

Bon appétit, dear reader. And may your vitality radiate like a thousand suns.

With warmth and gratitude,

Your Culinary Companion